How to Live with Gastroparesis

Guides, Tips, and Recipes to Relieve Gastroparesis.

Michael Samuel

TABLE OF CONTENTS

Part I: Understanding Gastroparesis

1. Introduction to Gastroparesis

What is Gastroparesis?

Gastroparesis is a medical condition characterized by delayed emptying of the stomach contents into the small intestine. This occurs when the stomach muscles fail to function properly, leading to slow or halted digestion. As a result, food remains in the stomach longer than normal, causing a variety of gastrointestinal symptoms and complications.

The term "gastroparesis" comes from the Greek words "gastro," meaning stomach, and "paresis," meaning paralysis. Although the stomach is not completely paralyzed, its motility is significantly impaired. This condition can vary in severity, with some individuals experiencing mild symptoms, while others endure debilitating effects that significantly impact their quality of life.

Causes and Risk Factors

The exact cause of gastroparesis is often difficult to pinpoint. However, several known factors and conditions can contribute to its development:

1. Diabetes: One of the most common causes of gastroparesis is diabetes, particularly when blood sugar levels are poorly controlled. High blood sugar can damage the vagus nerve, which controls the muscles of the stomach, leading to delayed gastric emptying.

2. Surgery: Surgical procedures on the stomach or nearby organs can damage the vagus nerve or other nerves involved in gastric motility, resulting in gastroparesis.

3. Medications: Certain medications, such as opioids, antidepressants, and medications used to treat high blood pressure, can interfere with stomach muscle contractions and slow gastric emptying.

4. Neurological Disorders: Conditions such as Parkinson's disease, multiple sclerosis, and other

neurological disorders can affect the nerves and muscles that control the stomach, leading to gastroparesis.

5. Infections: Viral infections, particularly involving the stomach or intestines, can sometimes trigger gastroparesis.

6. Autoimmune Diseases: Conditions like scleroderma or lupus can cause inflammation and damage to the stomach muscles or nerves, resulting in delayed gastric emptying.

7. Idiopathic Gastroparesis: In many cases, the cause of gastroparesis remains unknown. This is referred to as idiopathic gastroparesis.

Symptoms and Diagnosis

The symptoms of gastroparesis can vary widely in severity and frequency. Common symptoms include:

1. Nausea and Vomiting: These are often the most debilitating symptoms. Individuals with gastroparesis may feel persistently nauseous and may vomit undigested food hours after eating.

2. Bloating: A feeling of fullness or bloating in the stomach, even after eating only a small amount of food, is common.

3. Abdominal Pain: Some individuals experience pain or discomfort in the upper abdomen.

4. Early Satiety: Feeling full after eating only a small portion of food can be a significant issue, leading to inadequate nutrition.

5. Weight Loss and Malnutrition: Due to reduced food intake and poor absorption of nutrients, weight loss and malnutrition can occur.

6. Heartburn and Acid Reflux: Delayed stomach emptying can cause stomach acid to back up into the esophagus, leading to heartburn and acid reflux.

Diagnosis

Diagnosing gastroparesis typically involves a combination of medical history, physical examination, and specialized tests. Key diagnostic methods include:

1. Gastric Emptying Study: This is the most common test for diagnosing gastroparesis. The patient consumes a meal containing a small amount of radioactive material, and a scanner tracks how quickly the food leaves the stomach.

2. Upper Endoscopy: This procedure involves inserting a thin, flexible tube with a camera into the stomach to visually inspect the stomach lining and rule out other potential causes of symptoms.

3. SmartPill: This is a small, ingestible device that measures and records data on the gastrointestinal tract's motility as it passes through the digestive system.

4. Barium X-ray: The patient drinks a barium solution, and X-rays are taken to visualize the stomach and intestines. This test helps identify any blockages or structural abnormalities.

5. Electrogastrography: This test measures the electrical activity of the stomach muscles to detect abnormal rhythms.

6. Blood Tests: Blood tests may be conducted to check for underlying conditions such as diabetes or infections that could contribute to gastroparesis.

Understanding gastroparesis is the first step toward managing this challenging condition. With a proper diagnosis and a comprehensive treatment plan, individuals with gastroparesis can improve their quality of life and alleviate symptoms.

2. The Impact of Gastroparesis on Daily Life

Physical Effects

Gastroparesis significantly impacts the physical well-being of those affected. Some of the most notable physical effects include:

1. Nutritional Deficiencies: Due to prolonged gastric emptying, individuals may struggle to consume and absorb essential nutrients, leading to deficiencies. This can result in fatigue, weakened immune function, and poor overall health.

2. Dehydration: Persistent vomiting and nausea can lead to dehydration, which exacerbates feelings of fatigue and weakness.

3. Weight Loss: The inability to consume adequate calories due to early satiety and vomiting often results in unintended weight loss,

which can lead to muscle wasting and decreased physical strength.

4. Malnutrition: In severe cases, gastroparesis can cause malnutrition, where the body does not get enough vitamins and minerals. This can result in brittle bones, anemia, and a host of other health issues.

5. Digestive Discomfort: Symptoms such as bloating, abdominal pain, and acid reflux can cause significant discomfort and disrupt daily activities. Chronic discomfort may also lead to decreased appetite and further nutritional challenges.

Emotional and Mental Health

Living with a chronic condition like gastroparesis can take a toll on emotional and mental health:

1. Anxiety and Depression: The unpredictability of symptoms and the chronic nature of

gastroparesis can lead to anxiety and depression. Patients may feel overwhelmed by their condition and worried about their ability to manage daily activities.

2. Social Isolation: Due to the nature of their symptoms, individuals with gastroparesis might avoid social gatherings and eating out, leading to feelings of loneliness and isolation.

3. Stress: Constantly dealing with symptoms and managing dietary restrictions can be highly stressful. This stress can exacerbate physical symptoms, creating a vicious cycle.

4. Emotional Eating Challenges: Food is often associated with social activities and comfort. For those with gastroparesis, the need to follow a restricted diet can lead to frustration and a strained relationship with food.

5. Self-Esteem Issues: Weight fluctuations, physical discomfort, and dietary restrictions can

negatively impact self-esteem and body image, leading to further emotional distress.

Social and Professional Implications

The impact of gastroparesis extends beyond personal health, affecting social interactions and professional life:

1. Social Life: The need to adhere to a strict diet and the unpredictability of symptoms can make socializing difficult. Events centered around food, such as dinners and parties, can become sources of anxiety and discomfort, leading individuals to withdraw from social activities.

2. Relationships: Close relationships can be strained by the demands of managing gastroparesis. Loved ones may struggle to understand the condition, leading to misunderstandings and frustration on both sides.

3. Work and Productivity: Frequent symptoms like nausea, vomiting, and fatigue can interfere

with professional responsibilities. Individuals may need to take frequent breaks or sick leave, which can affect job performance and career advancement.

4. Financial Strain: Managing gastroparesis often involves significant medical expenses, including doctor visits, medications, and specialized diets. This can place a financial burden on individuals and their families.

5. Dietary Challenges: Eating out or traveling for work can be particularly challenging due to the need for specific, easily digestible foods. This can limit career opportunities and social interactions related to work.

Understanding the wide-ranging impact of gastroparesis on daily life highlights the importance of a comprehensive management approach. Addressing not only the physical symptoms but also the emotional, social, and professional challenges can significantly improve the quality of life for those living with this condition.

Part II:

Managing Gastroparesis

3. Medical Treatments and Interventions

Managing gastroparesis involves a combination of medical treatments and lifestyle adjustments to alleviate symptoms and improve quality of life. This section covers the primary medical treatments and interventions available.

Medications

Several medications can help manage the symptoms of gastroparesis by improving gastric motility and addressing specific symptoms such as nausea and vomiting. Commonly prescribed medications include:

1. Prokinetic Agents: These medications stimulate stomach muscle contractions to enhance gastric emptying.

- **Metoclopramide:** A commonly used prokinetic agent that increases muscle contractions in the upper digestive tract. It also has anti-nausea properties. However, long-term use can cause serious side effects, including tardive dyskinesia, a condition involving involuntary muscle movements.

- **Domperidone:** Similar to metoclopramide, domperidone enhances stomach contractions and reduces nausea. It is not available in the United States but can be obtained in other countries.

- **Erythromycin:** An antibiotic that, at lower doses, acts as a prokinetic agent by stimulating stomach motility. However, its effectiveness may diminish over time.

2. Antiemetic Medications: These drugs help control nausea and vomiting.

- **Ondansetron:** Commonly used to prevent nausea and vomiting, especially in patients undergoing chemotherapy.

- **Prochlorperazine:** Often prescribed to manage severe nausea and vomiting.

3. Antidepressants and Antianxiety **Medications:** Low doses of tricyclic antidepressants, such as amitriptyline, can help manage pain and discomfort associated with gastroparesis. Additionally, addressing anxiety can help reduce symptom severity.

4. Gastric Motility Agents:

 - **Bethanechol:** A cholinergic agent that stimulates muscle contractions in the stomach. Its usc is limited due to potential side effects.

Surgical Options

For individuals with severe gastroparesis who do not respond to medication, surgical interventions may be considered. These procedures aim to improve gastric emptying and alleviate symptoms.

1. Gastric Electrical Stimulation (GES): This procedure involves implanting a device that delivers mild electrical pulses to the stomach muscles. The stimulation helps improve gastric

motility and reduce nausea and vomiting. While GES can be effective, it is generally reserved for patients who have not responded to other treatments.

2. Pyloroplasty: This surgical procedure involves widening the pylorus, the opening between the stomach and the small intestine, to facilitate gastric emptying. Pyloroplasty can help reduce symptoms of gastroparesis, particularly in patients with a narrow pylorus.

3. Gastrojejunostomy: This procedure creates a direct connection between the stomach and the jejunum (a part of the small intestine), bypassing the pylorus. Gastrojejunostomy can improve gastric emptying and alleviate symptoms.

4. Gastrectomy: In extreme cases, partial or total removal of the stomach (gastrectomy) may be considered. This procedure is typically reserved for patients with severe, refractory gastroparesis and can significantly alter the digestive process.

Alternative Therapies

In addition to conventional medical treatments, several alternative therapies can help manage gastroparesis symptoms. These therapies are often used in conjunction with standard treatments to provide comprehensive symptom relief.

1. Dietary Modifications:
   - **Small, Frequent Meals:** Eating smaller meals more frequently throughout the day can help reduce the burden on the stomach and improve gastric emptying.
   - **Low-Fat, Low-Fiber Diet:** Foods high in fat and fiber can slow gastric emptying. A diet low in these components can help minimize symptoms.
   - **Pureed and Liquid Foods:** These are easier to digest and can be more comfortable for individuals with gastroparesis.

2. Nutritional Support: For patients who struggle to maintain adequate nutrition, enteral nutrition

(via feeding tube) or parenteral nutrition (intravenous feeding) may be necessary.

3. Acupuncture: Some studies suggest that acupuncture can help reduce symptoms of gastroparesis, such as nausea and vomiting, by stimulating specific points on the body.

4. Botulinum Toxin (Botox) Injections: Injecting Botox into the pyloric sphincter can relax the muscle and improve gastric emptying. This treatment is still considered experimental and its long-term effectiveness is uncertain.

5. Herbal and Natural Remedies: Some patients find relief with herbal supplements such as ginger, which has anti-nausea properties, or peppermint, which can help relax the gastrointestinal muscles. Always consult a healthcare provider before using herbal remedies.

6. Biofeedback and Relaxation Techniques: Stress management techniques, including

biofeedback, meditation, and deep breathing exercises, can help reduce the severity of symptoms by promoting relaxation and reducing anxiety.

7. Physical Therapy and Exercise: Regular, gentle exercise can stimulate gastric motility and help manage symptoms. Activities like walking after meals can be particularly beneficial.

Gastroparesis requires a multifaceted approach to management, tailored to the individual's specific needs and symptoms. By combining medical treatments, surgical options, and alternative therapies, patients can achieve better symptom control and improve their quality of life.

4. Dietary Management

Effective dietary management is crucial for individuals with gastroparesis. Proper nutrition helps maintain energy levels, prevents malnutrition, and can alleviate symptoms. This section explores the importance of nutrition, foods to avoid, and recommended foods and nutrients.

Importance of Nutrition

Nutrition plays a vital role in managing gastroparesis. The goals of dietary management are to:

1. Ensure Adequate Caloric Intake: Consuming enough calories is essential to prevent weight loss and maintain energy levels. Small, frequent meals can help achieve this without overwhelming the stomach.

2. Maintain Nutritional Balance: A well-balanced diet that includes all essential nutrients helps prevent deficiencies and supports overall health. This can be challenging with gastroparesis, so careful food choices are necessary.

3. Minimize Symptoms: Certain foods and eating habits can exacerbate symptoms like nausea, vomiting, and bloating. Adjusting the diet can help reduce these symptoms and improve quality of life.

Foods to Avoid

Certain foods can worsen gastroparesis symptoms by slowing gastric emptying or being difficult to digest. Avoiding these foods can help manage symptoms more effectively:

1. High-Fat Foods: Foods high in fat can delay gastric emptying and increase symptoms of bloating and nausea. Avoid fatty cuts of meat, fried foods, full-fat dairy products, and rich desserts.

2. High-Fiber Foods: Fiber is generally beneficial for digestion, but in gastroparesis, it can be problematic. Foods high in insoluble fiber are harder to digest and can cause blockages.

Avoid raw vegetables, whole grains, nuts, seeds, and legumes.

3. Tough Meats: Meats that are tough or have a lot of connective tissue can be hard to digest. Opt for tender cuts of meat or consider pureeing meat for easier consumption.

4. Carbonated Beverages: These can cause bloating and discomfort. Avoid soda, sparkling water, and other carbonated drinks.

5. Acidic Foods: Foods and beverages high in acid, such as citrus fruits, tomatoes, and coffee, can irritate the stomach lining and exacerbate symptoms.

6. Spicy Foods: Spices can irritate the stomach and worsen nausea and discomfort. Avoid heavily spiced dishes.

7. Alcohol: Alcohol can delay gastric emptying and irritate the stomach lining, leading to increased symptoms.

Recommended Foods and Nutrients

Choosing the right foods can help manage gastroparesis symptoms and ensure adequate nutrition. Here are some recommended foods and nutrients:

1. Low-Fat, Low-Fiber Foods: These are easier to digest and less likely to cause symptoms.

- **Lean Proteins:** Opt for lean cuts of poultry, fish, and tofu. Eggs and low-fat dairy products like yogurt and cottage cheese are also good options.

- **Refined Grains:** White rice, pasta, and white bread are easier to digest than whole grains. Consider fortified versions to increase nutrient intake.

- **Cooked Vegetables:** Cooking vegetables softens them, making them easier to digest. Carrots, green beans, and peeled potatoes are good choices.

- **Fruits:** Choose canned or cooked fruits without skins, such as applesauce, peaches, and pears. Bananas are also generally well-tolerated.

2. Pureed and Liquid Foods: These can be easier to manage and provide essential nutrients.
   - **Smoothies:** Blending fruits with low-fat yogurt or milk can create a nutritious and easy-to-digest meal. Add protein powder if needed.
   - **Soups and Broths:** Pureed soups made with low-fat ingredients can be soothing and nutritious.
   - **Meal Replacement Shakes:** These can be useful for ensuring adequate caloric and nutrient intake, especially during flare-ups.

3. Hydration: Staying hydrated is crucial, especially if vomiting is a concern.
   - **Water:** Sip water throughout the day to maintain hydration.
   - **Electrolyte Solutions:** These can help replace lost electrolytes if vomiting or diarrhea occurs.

4. Small, Frequent Meals: Eating smaller meals more frequently throughout the day can help manage symptoms and ensure adequate nutrition. Aim for five to six small meals instead of three large ones.

5. Healthy Fats: While high-fat foods should be limited, small amounts of healthy fats can be beneficial.
   - **Avocado:** This can be added in small quantities to meals for healthy fats.
   - **Olive Oil:** Use sparingly in cooking or dressings.

6. Supplements: Nutritional supplements may be necessary to ensure adequate intake of vitamins and minerals. Consult with a healthcare provider before starting any supplements.

Managing gastroparesis through dietary modifications requires careful planning and attention to individual tolerance. Working with a dietitian or nutritionist can help tailor a diet plan that meets nutritional needs while minimizing symptoms.

5. Lifestyle Adjustments

Effective management of gastroparesis extends beyond medical treatments and dietary changes. Lifestyle adjustments play a crucial role in minimizing symptoms and improving overall well-being. This section explores the importance of exercise, stress management techniques, and proper sleep and rest.

Exercise and Physical Activity

Regular exercise can significantly benefit individuals with gastroparesis by promoting overall health and enhancing digestive function. Here are some key points to consider:

1. Promoting Gastric Motility: Gentle physical activity can help stimulate stomach muscles and

promote gastric emptying. Activities like walking after meals can be particularly effective.

2. Choosing the Right Exercise: Low-impact exercises are generally well-tolerated and beneficial for those with gastroparesis. These include:
   - Walking: A simple and effective way to promote digestion and maintain fitness.
   - Yoga: Certain yoga poses can aid digestion and reduce stress, which can help manage symptoms.
   - Swimming: Provides a full-body workout without putting too much strain on the body.
   - Cycling: A gentle way to get cardiovascular exercise and promote overall health.

3. Timing of Exercise: It's best to engage in physical activity after meals rather than before. Walking for 15-30 minutes after eating can help with digestion and reduce symptoms.

4. Listening to Your Body: It's important to pay attention to how your body responds to exercise.

If any activity causes discomfort or exacerbates symptoms, it's best to stop and try a different form of exercise.

Stress Management Techniques

Stress can significantly impact the severity of gastroparesis symptoms. Implementing effective stress management techniques can help improve overall well-being and symptom control:

1. Mindfulness and Meditation: Practicing mindfulness and meditation can help reduce stress and anxiety. Techniques such as deep breathing, progressive muscle relaxation, and guided imagery can be beneficial.

2. Cognitive Behavioral Therapy (CBT): CBT is a structured, goal-oriented therapy that helps individuals identify and change negative thought patterns. It can be particularly effective in managing the anxiety and depression associated with chronic conditions like gastroparesis.

3. Physical Relaxation Techniques: Engaging in activities that promote relaxation can help manage stress. These include:

   - Massage Therapy: Can help relax muscles and reduce stress.

   - Aromatherapy: Using essential oils like lavender and chamomile can create a calming environment.

   - Tai Chi and Qi Gong: These gentle, flowing movements can reduce stress and improve overall well-being.

4. Social Support: Building a strong support network of friends, family, and support groups can provide emotional support and reduce feelings of isolation. Sharing experiences and coping strategies with others who understand the condition can be particularly comforting.

5. Hobbies and Leisure Activities: Engaging in activities that bring joy and relaxation can be a great way to manage stress. Whether it's reading, gardening, painting, or listening to music, finding time for leisure activities is important.

Sleep and Rest

Adequate sleep and rest are essential for managing gastroparesis and maintaining overall health. Here are some tips to ensure quality sleep and rest:

1. Establish a Regular Sleep Routine: Going to bed and waking up at the same time each day helps regulate the body's internal clock and improve sleep quality.

2. Create a Restful Environment: Make sure the sleep environment is conducive to rest. This includes a comfortable mattress, a dark and quiet room, and a cool temperature.

3. Avoid Heavy Meals Before Bedtime: Eating large meals close to bedtime can exacerbate symptoms and interfere with sleep. Aim to finish eating at least 2-3 hours before going to bed.

4. Limit Stimulants: Avoid caffeine and nicotine in the evening, as they can disrupt sleep patterns.

5. Practice Relaxation Techniques Before Bed: Engage in calming activities before bedtime, such as reading a book, taking a warm bath, or practicing relaxation exercises.

6. Manage Nighttime Symptoms: If symptoms like nausea or acid reflux occur at night, try elevating the head of the bed or using additional pillows to keep the upper body elevated.

7. Seek Professional Help if Needed: If sleep disturbances are severe or persistent, consider seeking help from a healthcare provider or a sleep specialist.

Incorporating these lifestyle adjustments can help individuals with gastroparesis manage their symptoms more effectively and improve their overall quality of life. Balancing physical activity, stress management, and proper rest is essential for maintaining health and well-being.

6. Monitoring and Tracking Symptoms

Effectively managing gastroparesis involves consistent monitoring and tracking of symptoms to identify patterns, triggers, and the effectiveness of treatments. This section discusses the importance of keeping a symptom diary, recognizing triggers, and maintaining regular check-ups with healthcare providers.

Keeping a Symptom Diary

A symptom diary is an essential tool for individuals with gastroparesis. It helps track the frequency, severity, and context of symptoms, providing valuable insights for both patients and healthcare providers.

1. Recording Symptoms: Note the type of symptoms experienced (e.g., nausea, vomiting,

bloating, pain), their intensity, and duration. Use a scale (e.g., 1-10) to rate symptom severity.

2. Tracking Meals: Document what foods were eaten, the portion sizes, and the timing of meals. Include details about any beverages consumed.

3. Medication and Treatment: Keep track of any medications or treatments taken, including the dosage and time of administration. Note any changes in symptoms after taking medication.

4. Physical Activity: Record any physical activities performed, their duration, and intensity. Note if there were any changes in symptoms post-exercise.

5. Emotional and Mental Health: Include notes about stress levels, mood, and any significant emotional events. This can help identify if stress or emotional factors are contributing to symptom flare-ups.

6. Bowel Movements: Record details about bowel movements, including frequency, consistency, and any difficulties experienced.

Recognizing Triggers

Identifying and understanding triggers is crucial for managing gastroparesis. A symptom diary can help recognize patterns and pinpoint specific factors that exacerbate symptoms.

1. Dietary Triggers: Certain foods or beverages may consistently lead to symptom flare-ups. Common dietary triggers include high-fat foods, high-fiber foods, and carbonated beverages.

2. Lifestyle Triggers: Activities such as vigorous exercise, stress, or inadequate sleep may worsen symptoms. Identifying these lifestyle triggers allows for better management and adjustment of daily routines.

3. Medication Triggers: Some medications may contribute to gastroparesis symptoms. Keeping

track of medication intake and corresponding symptoms can help identify problematic drugs.

4. Environmental Triggers: Changes in environment, such as traveling, extreme weather conditions, or exposure to allergens, may impact symptoms.

Regular Check-Ups with Healthcare Providers

Consistent communication with healthcare providers is essential for effective management of gastroparesis. Regular check-ups ensure that treatment plans are up-to-date and adjusted as needed.

1. Routine Appointments: Schedule regular visits with your primary care physician and gastroenterologist. These appointments help monitor the progression of the condition and make necessary adjustments to treatment plans.

2. Sharing Symptom Diary: Bring your symptom diary to appointments. This detailed record helps healthcare providers understand your condition better and make informed decisions about your treatment.

3. Nutritional Counseling: Regular visits with a dietitian or nutritionist can help ensure you are meeting your nutritional needs while managing symptoms. They can provide personalized dietary recommendations and adjustments.

4. Mental Health Support: Consider regular check-ins with a mental health professional, especially if you are experiencing anxiety or depression related to gastroparesis. They can provide coping strategies and support.

5. Monitoring Medication and Treatments: Regular check-ups allow healthcare providers to monitor the effectiveness of medications and treatments. They can adjust dosages, prescribe new medications, or recommend alternative therapies as needed.

6. Screening for Complications: Gastroparesis can lead to complications such as malnutrition, dehydration, and severe weight loss. Regular check-ups help in early detection and management of these complications.

7. Education and Support: Healthcare providers can offer education about gastroparesis, new treatments, and research developments. They can also connect you with support groups and resources for additional assistance.

By diligently monitoring symptoms, recognizing triggers, and maintaining regular check-ups with healthcare providers, individuals with gastroparesis can achieve better symptom control and improve their overall quality of life. This proactive approach allows for timely adjustments to treatment plans and helps prevent complications.

Part III: Recipes for Gastroparesis Relief

7. Breakfast Ideas

Starting the day with a nutritious and easy-to-digest breakfast can set a positive tone for managing gastroparesis symptoms. This section provides recipes and ideas for smoothies, shakes, and soft, easy-to-digest breakfasts.

Smoothies and Shakes

Smoothies and shakes are excellent options for individuals with gastroparesis as they are easy to prepare, nutrient-dense, and gentle on the stomach. Here are some delicious and soothing recipes:

1. Banana Almond Smoothie
  - **Ingredients:**
    - 1 ripe banana

- 1 cup almond milk (or other low-fat milk alternatives)
    - 1 tablespoon almond butter
    - 1 tablespoon honey or maple syrup
    - 1/2 teaspoon vanilla extract
  - **Instructions:**
    1. Combine all ingredients in a blender.
    2. Blend until smooth and creamy.
    3. Serve immediately.

2. Peach Yogurt Smoothie
  - **Ingredients:**
    - 1 cup canned peaches (drained and rinsed)
    - 1/2 cup low-fat yogurt
    - 1/2 cup orange juice (or other fruit juice)
    - 1 tablespoon honey
  - **Instructions:**
    1. Place all ingredients in a blender.
    2. Blend until smooth.
    3. Pour into a glass and enjoy.

3. Berry Protein Shake
  - **Ingredients:**
    - 1/2 cup mixed berries (fresh or frozen)

- 1 scoop protein powder (vanilla or unflavored)
    - 1 cup low-fat milk or milk alternative
    - 1 tablespoon flaxseed oil or chia seeds
    - 1/2 teaspoon vanilla extract
- **Instructions:**
    1. Add all ingredients to a blender.
    2. Blend until thoroughly mixed and smooth.
    3. Serve chilled.

4. Oatmeal Banana Smoothie
- **Ingredients:**
    - 1/2 cup cooked oatmeal
    - 1 ripe banana
    - 1 cup almond milk or low-fat milk
    - 1 tablespoon honey
    - 1/2 teaspoon cinnamon
- **Instructions:**
    1. Combine all ingredients in a blender.
    2. Blend until smooth and creamy.
    3. Pour into a glass and enjoy.

Soft and Easy-to-Digest Breakfasts

These breakfast ideas are designed to be gentle on the stomach while providing essential nutrients.

1. Scrambled Eggs with Spinach
- **Ingredients:**
  - 2 eggs
  - 1/4 cup low-fat milk
  - 1/4 cup cooked spinach (well-drained)
  - Salt and pepper to taste
  - 1 teaspoon olive oil
- **Instructions:**
  1. Beat eggs and milk together in a bowl.
  2. Heat olive oil in a non-stick skillet over medium heat.
  3. Pour egg mixture into the skillet and cook, stirring gently, until eggs are almost set.
  4. Add spinach and cook until eggs are fully set.
  5. Season with salt and pepper and serve.

2. Creamy Rice Pudding
- **Ingredients:**
  - 1/2 cup cooked white rice

- 1 cup low-fat milk
- 1 tablespoon sugar or honey
- 1/2 teaspoon vanilla extract
- Ground cinnamon for garnish
  - **Instructions:**

1. Combine cooked rice, milk, sugar, and vanilla in a saucepan.

2. Cook over medium heat, stirring frequently, until the mixture thickens and becomes creamy.

3. Serve warm, sprinkled with a pinch of cinnamon.

3. Applesauce Pancakes
  - **Ingredients:**
    - 1 cup all-purpose flour
    - 1 tablespoon sugar
    - 1 teaspoon baking powder
    - 1/2 teaspoon baking soda
    - 1/4 teaspoon salt
    - 1 cup applesauce
    - 1/2 cup low-fat milk
    - 1 egg
    - 1 teaspoon vanilla extract

- 1 tablespoon vegetable oil
- **Instructions:**
1. In a bowl, whisk together flour, sugar, baking powder, baking soda, and salt.
2. In another bowl, mix applesauce, milk, egg, vanilla, and oil.
3. Pour the wet ingredients into the dry ingredients and stir until just combined.
4. Heat a non-stick skillet over medium heat and lightly grease it.
5. Pour 1/4 cup of batter for each pancake onto the skillet and cook until bubbles form on the surface. Flip and cook until golden brown.
6. Serve warm with a drizzle of maple syrup or honey.

4. Cottage Cheese with Soft Fruits
  - **Ingredients:**
    - 1 cup low-fat cottage cheese
    - 1/2 cup canned or cooked fruit (such as peaches, pears, or apples)
    - 1 tablespoon honey or maple syrup
    - Ground cinnamon for garnish (optional)
  - **Instructions:**

1. Scoop cottage cheese into a bowl.

2. Top with fruit and drizzle with honey or maple syrup.

3. Sprinkle with cinnamon if desired and serve.

5. Overnight Oats
   - **Ingredients:**
     - 1/2 cup rolled oats
     - 1 cup low-fat milk or milk alternative
     - 1/2 cup low-fat yogurt
     - 1 tablespoon honey
     - 1/4 cup soft fruit (such as berries or banana slices)
   - **Instructions:**
     1. Combine oats, milk, yogurt, and honey in a jar or container.

     2. Stir well and cover.

     3. Refrigerate overnight.

     4. In the morning, top with soft fruit and enjoy.

These breakfast ideas provide a variety of options that are easy on the stomach while still being nutritious and satisfying. Adjust ingredients and portions to meet individual tolerances and preferences.

8. Lunch and Dinner Recipes

When managing gastroparesis, it's essential to focus on meals that are light, nutritious, and easy to digest. This section offers a variety of recipes for soups, main courses, side dishes, and snacks that are designed to be gentle on the stomach while providing essential nutrients.

Light and Nutritious Soups

1. Creamy Carrot Ginger Soup
  - Ingredients:
    - 1 pound carrots, peeled and sliced
    - 1 small onion, chopped
    - 1 tablespoon olive oil
    - 1 teaspoon grated fresh ginger
    - 4 cups low-sodium vegetable broth
    - 1/2 cup low-fat milk or cream

- Salt and pepper to taste

- Instructions:

1. In a large pot, heat olive oil over medium heat.

2. Add chopped onion and cook until soft, about 5 minutes.

3. Add carrots and ginger, and cook for another 5 minutes.

4. Pour in vegetable broth and bring to a boil.

5. Reduce heat and simmer until carrots are tender, about 20 minutes.

6. Puree the soup using an immersion blender or in batches in a regular blender until smooth.

7. Stir in milk or cream, and season with salt and pepper.

8. Serve warm.

2. Chicken and Rice Soup

- Ingredients:

- 1 cup cooked, shredded chicken breast
- 1/2 cup cooked white rice
- 1 small carrot, peeled and diced
- 1 small potato, peeled and diced
- 4 cups low-sodium chicken broth

- 1 tablespoon olive oil

- Salt and pepper to taste

- Instructions:

1. In a large pot, heat olive oil over medium heat.

2. Add diced carrot and potato, and cook until softened, about 5 minutes.

3. Pour in chicken broth and bring to a boil.

4. Reduce heat and simmer until vegetables are tender, about 15 minutes.

5. Stir in cooked chicken and rice, and season with salt and pepper.

6. Cook for an additional 5 minutes, until heated through.

7. Serve warm.

3. Butternut Squash Soup

- Ingredients:

- 1 medium butternut squash, peeled, seeded, and cubed

- 1 small onion, chopped

- 1 tablespoon olive oil

- 4 cups low-sodium vegetable broth

- 1/2 cup low-fat milk or cream

- Salt and pepper to taste

- Instructions:

1. In a large pot, heat olive oil over medium heat.

2. Add chopped onion and cook until soft, about 5 minutes.

3. Add butternut squash and vegetable broth, and bring to a boil.

4. Reduce heat and simmer until squash is tender, about 20 minutes.

5. Puree the soup using an immersion blender or in batches in a regular blender until smooth.

6. Stir in milk or cream, and season with salt and pepper.

7. Serve warm.

Easily Digestible Main Courses

1. Baked Cod with Lemon and Herbs
   - Ingredients:
   - 4 cod fillets
   - 2 tablespoons olive oil
   - 1 lemon, thinly sliced
   - 1 teaspoon dried thyme

- 1 teaspoon dried oregano
- Salt and pepper to taste
- Instructions:

1. Preheat oven to 375°F (190°C).

2. Place cod fillets in a baking dish.

3. Drizzle with olive oil and season with thyme, oregano, salt, and pepper.

4. Arrange lemon slices on top of the fillets.

5. Bake for 15-20 minutes, until fish is opaque and flakes easily with a fork.

6. Serve with a side of steamed vegetables.

2. Chicken and Vegetable Stir-Fry

- Ingredients:

- 2 boneless, skinless chicken breasts, thinly sliced
- 1 cup broccoli florets
- 1 small zucchini, sliced
- 1 small bell pepper, sliced
- 1 tablespoon olive oil
- 2 tablespoons low-sodium soy sauce
- 1 teaspoon grated fresh ginger
- 1 clove garlic, minced

- Instructions:

1. In a large skillet, heat olive oil over medium-high heat.

2. Add chicken slices and cook until no longer pink, about 5 minutes.

3. Add broccoli, zucchini, and bell pepper, and cook until vegetables are tender, about 5-7 minutes.

4. Stir in soy sauce, ginger, and garlic, and cook for an additional 2 minutes.

5. Serve warm with steamed rice or quinoa.

3. Turkey Meatballs with Mashed Potatoes

- Ingredients:
- 1 pound ground turkey
- 1/4 cup breadcrumbs
- 1 egg, beaten
- 1/4 cup grated Parmesan cheese
- 1 teaspoon dried parsley
- Salt and pepper to taste
- 4 large potatoes, peeled and cubed
- 1/2 cup low-fat milk
- 2 tablespoons butter

- Instructions:
1. Preheat oven to 375°F (190°C).

2. In a bowl, combine ground turkey, breadcrumbs, egg, Parmesan cheese, parsley, salt, and pepper. Mix well.

3. Form mixture into meatballs and place on a baking sheet.

4. Bake for 20-25 minutes, until meatballs are cooked through.

5. Meanwhile, cook potatoes in boiling water until tender, about 15 minutes.

6. Drain and mash with milk and butter until smooth.

7. Serve meatballs over mashed potatoes.

Side Dishes and Snacks

1. Steamed Green Beans with Lemon
  - Ingredients:
    - 1 pound green beans, trimmed
    - 1 tablespoon olive oil
    - Juice of 1 lemon
    - Salt and pepper to taste
  - Instructions:
    1. Steam green beans until tender, about 5-7 minutes.

2. Toss with olive oil, lemon juice, salt, and pepper.

3. Serve warm.

2. Mashed Sweet Potatoes

- Ingredients:
- 2 large sweet potatoes, peeled and cubed
- 1/2 cup low-fat milk
- 2 tablespoons butter
- 1 tablespoon maple syrup
- Salt to taste

- Instructions:
1. Boil sweet potatoes until tender, about 15 minutes.

2. Drain and mash with milk, butter, and maple syrup.

3. Season with salt and serve warm.

3. Cottage Cheese and Fruit Snack

- Ingredients:
- 1 cup low-fat cottage cheese
- 1/2 cup canned fruit (peaches, pears, or mandarin oranges)
- 1 tablespoon honey or maple syrup

- Instructions:

1. Scoop cottage cheese into a bowl.

2. Top with fruit and drizzle with honey or maple syrup.

3. Serve as a light snack.

4. Banana Rice Pudding

- Ingredients:

- 1/2 cup cooked white rice
- 1 cup low-fat milk
- 1 ripe banana, mashed
- 1 tablespoon honey
- 1/2 teaspoon vanilla extract

- Instructions:

1. Combine cooked rice, milk, mashed banana, honey, and vanilla in a saucepan.

2. Cook over medium heat, stirring frequently, until the mixture thickens.

3. Serve warm or chilled.

These recipes provide a variety of lunch and dinner options that are gentle on the stomach, nutritious, and satisfying. Adjust ingredients and portion sizes based on individual tolerance and nutritional needs.

9. Snacks and Beverages

Choosing appropriate snacks and beverages can help manage gastroparesis symptoms while providing necessary nutrients and hydration. This section offers ideas for healthy snacks and hydrating, nourishing drinks.

Healthy Snacks

1. Apple Slices with Almond Butter
  - **Ingredients:**
    - 1 apple, sliced
    - 2 tablespoons almond butter
  - **Instructions:**
    1. Spread almond butter on apple slices.
    2. Serve immediately.

2. Greek Yogurt with Honey and Soft Fruit
  - **Ingredients:**

- 1 cup plain Greek yogurt
- 1 tablespoon honey
- 1/2 cup soft fruit (e.g., canned peaches or berries)
  - **Instructions:**
    1. Mix Greek yogurt with honey.
    2. Top with soft fruit and serve.

3. Rice Cakes with Cottage Cheese
  - **Ingredients:**
    - 2 rice cakes
    - 1/2 cup low-fat cottage cheese
  - **Instructions:**
    1. Spread cottage cheese on rice cakes.
    2. Serve as a light snack.

4. Oatmeal Energy Balls
  - **Ingredients:**
    - 1 cup rolled oats
    - 1/4 cup honey
    - 1/4 cup almond butter
    - 1/4 cup mini chocolate chips (optional)
  - **Instructions:**
    1. Combine all ingredients in a bowl.

2. Roll mixture into small balls.

3. Store in an airtight container.

5. Mashed Avocado on Soft Bread
  - **Ingredients:**
    - 1 ripe avocado
    - 1-2 slices of soft, white bread
    - Salt to taste
  - **Instructions:**
    1. Mash avocado with a fork.
    2. Spread on soft bread.
    3. Season with a pinch of salt if desired.

Hydrating and Nourishing Drinks

1. Herbal Teas
  - **Ingredients:**
    - 1 herbal tea bag (e.g., chamomile or ginger)
    - 1 cup hot water
  - **Instructions:**
    1. Steep tea bag in hot water for 5 minutes.
    2. Remove tea bag and let cool slightly before drinking.

2. Coconut Water
  - **Ingredients:**
    - 1 cup coconut water (plain, unsweetened)
  - **Instructions:**
    1. Chill coconut water if desired.
    2. Serve cold for hydration.

3. Smoothie Popsicles
  - **Ingredients:**
    - 1 cup fruit juice (e.g., apple or pear)
    - 1/2 cup plain yogurt
    - 1/2 cup soft fruit (e.g., bananas or berries)
  - **Instructions:**
    1. Blend fruit juice, yogurt, and soft fruit until smooth.
    2. Pour into popsicle molds and freeze.
    3. Enjoy a refreshing, cold treat.

4. Rice Milk
  - **Ingredients:**
    - 1 cup rice milk
  - **Instructions:**
    1. Chill rice milk if desired.
    2. Serve cold or at room temperature.

5. Ginger Ale
  - **Ingredients:**
    - 1 cup ginger ale (plain or low-sugar)
  - **Instructions:**
    1. Chill ginger ale if desired.
    2. Serve cold for a soothing drink.

These snacks and beverages offer easy-to-digest options and hydration, helping to manage gastroparesis symptoms while keeping you nourished. Adjust the choices based on individual preferences and tolerances.

10. Desserts and Treats

Indulging in desserts and treats while managing gastroparesis requires careful selection of low-fat, low-fiber options that are easy to digest. This section provides recipes for satisfying sweets and tips for enjoying desserts safely.

Low-Fat and Low-Fiber Sweets

1. Baked Apples

- **Ingredients:**
  - 4 apples, cored
  - 1/4 cup honey
  - 1/4 teaspoon ground cinnamon
  - 1/4 cup water

- **Instructions:**
  1. Preheat oven to 350°F (175°C).
  2. Place apples in a baking dish.
  3. Drizzle with honey and sprinkle with cinnamon.
  4. Add water to the dish to help steam the apples.
  5. Bake for 20-25 minutes, until apples are tender.
  6. Serve warm.

2. Vanilla Pudding

- **Ingredients:**
  - 2 cups low-fat milk
  - 1/4 cup cornstarch
  - 1/4 cup sugar
  - 1 teaspoon vanilla extract

- Instructions:

1. In a saucepan, whisk together milk, cornstarch, and sugar.

2. Cook over medium heat, stirring constantly, until mixture thickens and starts to bubble.

3. Remove from heat and stir in vanilla extract.

4. Pour into serving dishes and let cool.

3. Banana Ice Cream

- Ingredients:

- 2 ripe bananas, peeled and sliced
- 1/4 cup low-fat milk or milk alternative

- Instructions:

1. Freeze banana slices for at least 2 hours.

2. Blend frozen bananas and milk until smooth and creamy.

3. Serve immediately or freeze for a firmer texture.

4. Rice Pudding

- Ingredients:

- 1/2 cup cooked white rice

- 1 cup low-fat milk
- 2 tablespoons sugar
- 1/4 teaspoon vanilla extract

- Instructions:

1. In a saucepan, combine rice, milk, and sugar.

2. Cook over medium heat, stirring frequently, until the mixture thickens.

3. Remove from heat and stir in vanilla extract.

4. Serve warm or chilled.

5. Peach Sorbet

- Ingredients:

- 2 cups canned peaches (drained)
- 1/4 cup sugar
- 1/2 cup water

- Instructions:

1. Blend peaches, sugar, and water until smooth.

2. Pour mixture into a shallow dish and freeze, stirring every 30 minutes until firm.

3. Serve scoops of sorbet as a refreshing treat.

Tips for Enjoying Desserts with Gastroparesis

1. Choose Low-Fat Options: Opt for desserts that use low-fat dairy products or alternatives to reduce fat intake, which can be easier on the digestive system.

2. Minimize Fiber: Select desserts that are low in fiber to avoid triggering symptoms. Avoid high-fiber ingredients like whole grains, nuts, and seeds.

3. Watch Portion Sizes: Small portions can help manage symptoms by preventing overloading the stomach. Enjoy desserts in moderation to avoid discomfort.

4. Avoid Rich or Creamy Desserts: Rich or overly creamy desserts can be harder to digest. Opt for lighter, simpler options that are easier on the stomach.

5. Consider Temperature: Some people with gastroparesis may find cold or frozen desserts

easier to tolerate. Experiment with different temperatures to see what works best.

6. Monitor Sugar Intake: While sweets can be a nice treat, excessive sugar may cause discomfort. Use natural sweeteners in moderation and balance with other nutrients.

7. Test Tolerances: Individual tolerances can vary, so try different dessert recipes to determine which ones work best for you. Keep a food diary to track how different sweets affect your symptoms.

By focusing on low-fat, low-fiber options and following these tips, you can enjoy delicious desserts while managing gastroparesis symptoms effectively.

Part IV:

Tips and Strategies for Daily Living

11. Eating Out and Socializing

Managing gastroparesis while eating out and participating in social events can be challenging but manageable with the right strategies. This section provides tips for choosing suitable restaurants and navigating social situations to ensure a comfortable dining experience.

Choosing Gastroparesis-Friendly Restaurants

1. Research Ahead:
   - Look up restaurants online to check their menus and see if they offer dishes that align with gastroparesis-friendly guidelines.
   - Call ahead to ask about the availability of specific items or to make special requests.

2. Look for Simple Menus:

- Choose restaurants that offer simple, straightforward dishes with minimal ingredients.

- Opt for places that serve grilled, baked, or steamed dishes instead of fried or heavily seasoned options.

3. Request Customizations:

- Don't hesitate to ask for modifications such as low-fat cooking methods, no added spices, or substitutions like plain rice instead of high-fiber sides.

- Request sauces and dressings on the side to control the amount used.

4. Avoid Buffets:

- Buffets can be challenging because they offer many high-fat or high-fiber options. It may be difficult to find suitable choices.

5. Check for Smaller Portions:

- Some restaurants offer smaller or "lite" portions which can be helpful in managing meal sizes and preventing overloading the stomach.

6. Ask About Ingredients:
- Inquire about the ingredients in dishes to avoid high-fiber or high-fat components. Clarify how dishes are prepared to ensure they meet your dietary needs.

Navigating Social Events and Gatherings

1. Plan Ahead:
- If possible, find out what food will be served at the event in advance and plan accordingly. If needed, bring your own dish that meets your dietary needs.

2. Eat Beforehand:
- Have a light, gastroparesis-friendly meal before attending the event to avoid hunger and reduce the temptation to eat foods that might trigger symptoms.

3. Communicate Your Needs:

   - Let hosts or event organizers know about your dietary restrictions politely. Most people will understand and may accommodate your needs.

4. Choose Safe Options:

   - At gatherings, focus on foods that you know are safe for you to eat. Stick to easily digestible options like plain proteins, steamed vegetables, and simple carbohydrates.

5. Be Mindful of Portions:

   - Serve yourself smaller portions to avoid overeating. You can always go back for more if you're still hungry and if your stomach feels up to it.

6. Stay Hydrated:

   - Drink water or suitable beverages to stay hydrated and aid digestion. Avoid high-sugar or caffeinated drinks which might irritate your stomach.

7. Know Your Limits:

  - If you're feeling unwell or overwhelmed, it's okay to excuse yourself from eating or leave the event early. Your comfort is a priority.

8. Be Honest About Your Needs:

  - If asked about your dietary choices, be honest about your need for specific foods. Sharing your situation can help others understand and provide support.

By implementing these tips, you can navigate dining out and social events with greater ease while managing gastroparesis. Preparing in advance and making informed choices can help you enjoy social interactions and meals more comfortably.

12. Traveling with Gastroparesis

Traveling with gastroparesis requires careful planning to ensure comfort and manage symptoms effectively. This section offers strategies for preparing for trips and handling symptoms while away from home.

Preparing for Trips

1. Plan Ahead:
   - Research your destination to find nearby grocery stores, pharmacies, and restaurants that offer gastroparesis-friendly options.
   - Make a list of necessary items to bring, including any medications and specialized foods.

2. Pack Smart:
   - Bring a variety of easy-to-digest snacks and meals that you know work well for you.
   - Pack medications in their original containers and carry a sufficient supply.

3. Create a Meal Plan:
   - Plan your meals and snacks ahead of time. Consider how you will manage eating in different settings, whether it's bringing your own food or finding suitable options.

4. Carry Important Documents:
   - Have a copy of your medical records, including a list of your medications and any relevant dietary information.
   - If traveling internationally, ensure you have any necessary prescriptions and understand local regulations regarding medication.

5. Contact Your Accommodation:
   - Inform your hotel or rental about your dietary needs. Request a room with a kitchenette if possible, so you can prepare your own meals.

6. Check Travel Insurance:
   - Ensure your travel insurance covers medical needs and includes coverage for any potential gastroparesis-related issues.

Managing Symptoms While Away

1. Stick to Your Routine:
   - Try to maintain your regular eating schedule and portion sizes as much as possible to keep symptoms under control.

2. Choose Safe Foods:
  - Stick to familiar, safe foods that you know are easy on your digestive system. Opt for bland, low-fat, and low-fiber options when dining out.

3. Stay Hydrated:
  - Drink plenty of water and suitable beverages to stay hydrated, especially if traveling to a different climate or altitude.

4. Monitor Symptoms:
  - Keep track of any changes in your symptoms or digestive responses. If you notice any significant issues, adjust your food choices or consult a local healthcare provider if needed.

5. Be Flexible:
  - Be prepared to adapt your plans if necessary. If you're unable to find suitable food options, consider eating smaller amounts more frequently to manage symptoms.

6. Rest and Relax:

- Ensure you get enough rest and manage stress to prevent exacerbating symptoms. Take breaks and avoid overexertion.

7. Know Local Healthcare Options:
   - Familiarize yourself with local healthcare facilities in case you need medical assistance. Keep contact information for local doctors or hospitals handy.

8. Communicate Your Needs:
   - Be open about your dietary restrictions when interacting with others. Most people will be understanding and supportive of your needs.

By planning ahead and staying adaptable, you can manage gastroparesis effectively while traveling, allowing you to enjoy your trip with fewer worries.

13. Building a Support System

A strong support system is crucial for managing gastroparesis effectively. It helps to have people who understand your condition and can provide emotional, practical, and informational support. This section provides guidance on finding support groups and communicating with friends and family.

Finding Support Groups

1. Online Communities:
   - Social Media: Join groups or forums on platforms like Facebook, Reddit, or specialized health forums where people with gastroparesis share their experiences and advice.
   - Support Websites: Look for websites dedicated to gastroparesis or chronic illness support. They often have forums or chat rooms for connecting with others.

2. Local Support Groups:
   - Hospitals and Clinics: Check with local hospitals, clinics, or gastroenterology offices for

information about local support groups or patient advocacy organizations.

- Community Centers: Many community centers or libraries host health-related support groups or can provide information about them.

3. Nonprofit Organizations:

- Gastroparesis Foundations: Organizations such as the Gastroparesis Support Network or other gastroparesis-specific foundations may offer support groups, resources, and events.

- Chronic Illness Networks: Explore general chronic illness or digestive health organizations that may have gastroparesis resources.

4. Medical Professionals:

- Doctors and Dietitians: Ask your healthcare providers for recommendations on support groups or resources where you can connect with others who have gastroparesis.

Communicating with Friends and Family

1. Educate Them:

- Share Information: Provide your friends and family with educational materials about gastroparesis so they understand the condition and its impact on your life.

- Explain Your Needs: Clearly communicate what you need from them, whether it's help with meal preparation, understanding your dietary restrictions, or just emotional support.

2. Set Boundaries:

- Be Honest: Explain any limitations or adjustments you need to make in your daily life. Let them know if you need time to rest or if certain activities may be challenging for you.

- Manage Expectations: Help your loved ones understand your limitations and adjust their expectations accordingly.

3. Seek Their Support:

- Ask for Help: Don't hesitate to ask for assistance with tasks that may be difficult due to your condition, such as cooking or grocery shopping.

- Involve Them in Your Care: Include them in your healthcare journey by discussing treatment plans, dietary changes, and symptom management.

4. Maintain Open Communication:
   - Regular Updates: Keep your friends and family informed about any changes in your condition or treatment. Regular updates help them understand your situation better.
   - Express Appreciation: Acknowledge and thank them for their support and understanding. Positive reinforcement can strengthen your relationships and support system.

5. Engage in Supportive Activities:
   - Shared Experiences: Involve your loved ones in activities that accommodate your condition, such as cooking gastroparesis-friendly meals together or participating in low-impact activities.
   - Emotional Support: Encourage open conversations about your feelings and experiences. Share both the challenges and successes to build empathy and understanding.

Building a robust support system involves connecting with others who understand and support your needs and communicating openly with friends and family. By fostering these relationships, you can enhance your well-being and manage gastroparesis more effectively.

14. Self-Care and Mental Well-being

Managing gastroparesis involves not only addressing physical symptoms but also taking care of your mental and emotional health. This section provides strategies for incorporating mindfulness and meditation into your routine and coping with anxiety and depression.

Mindfulness and Meditation

1. Mindfulness Practices:
   - Daily Mindfulness: Integrate mindfulness into your daily routine by paying attention to the present moment. This can be as simple as

focusing on your breath, observing your surroundings, or being fully engaged in daily activities.

   - Mindful Eating: Practice mindful eating by slowing down and savoring each bite. Pay attention to the textures, flavors, and sensations of your food to enhance your eating experience and improve digestion.

2. Meditation Techniques:

   - Guided Meditation: Use apps or online resources for guided meditations. These can help you relax and focus, reducing stress and improving overall well-being.

   - Breathing Exercises: Practice deep breathing exercises to calm your mind and body. Techniques like diaphragmatic breathing or the 4-7-8 method can help reduce anxiety and promote relaxation.

   - Progressive Muscle Relaxation: This technique involves tensing and then relaxing different muscle groups in your body to alleviate physical and mental tension.

3. Establish a Routine:

   - Consistency: Dedicate a specific time each day for mindfulness or meditation practice. Consistent practice can enhance its benefits and integrate it into your lifestyle more effectively.

   - Create a Calm Space: Set up a designated area for mindfulness and meditation that is quiet and free from distractions to help you focus and relax.

Coping with Anxiety and Depression

1. Recognize Symptoms:

   - Identify Triggers: Pay attention to situations or thoughts that trigger anxiety or depressive feelings. Understanding your triggers can help you address them more effectively.

   - Monitor Mood: Keep a journal to track your mood and symptoms. This can help you identify patterns and seek appropriate help if needed.

2. Seek Professional Help:

   - Therapy: Consider speaking with a mental health professional, such as a therapist or counselor, who can provide support and coping strategies for managing anxiety and depression.

- Medication: If necessary, consult with a healthcare provider about medications that may help alleviate symptoms of anxiety or depression.

3. Build a Support Network:

- Reach Out: Connect with friends, family, or support groups to share your feelings and experiences. Social support can provide comfort and understanding.

- Participate in Support Groups: Join support groups for individuals with chronic illnesses or mental health challenges. Sharing experiences and advice with others in similar situations can be beneficial.

4. Engage in Self-Care Activities:

- Physical Activity: Incorporate regular, gentle exercise into your routine, such as walking or stretching, to boost your mood and reduce stress.

- Hobbies and Interests: Engage in activities that you enjoy and that bring you satisfaction, whether it's reading, crafting, or spending time in nature.

5. Practice Self-Compassion:
   - Be Kind to Yourself: Acknowledge your efforts and challenges without self-judgment. Practice self-compassion by treating yourself with the same kindness and understanding you would offer to a friend.
   - Set Realistic Goals: Set achievable goals and be gentle with yourself if you face setbacks. Celebrate small victories and progress.

6. Develop Coping Strategies:
   - Stress Management: Use stress management techniques, such as time management, relaxation exercises, and healthy coping mechanisms, to handle daily stressors.
   - Positive Affirmations: Practice using positive affirmations to challenge negative thoughts and reinforce a positive mindset.

Taking care of your mental well-being through mindfulness, meditation, and effective coping strategies is essential for managing gastroparesis and improving your overall quality of life. By addressing both physical and emotional needs, you can create a balanced approach to self-care.

Part V:

Personal Stories and Experiences

15. Living with Gastroparesis: Real-Life Stories

Hearing from others who are living with gastroparesis can provide valuable insights, encouragement, and practical advice. This section features testimonials from gastroparesis patients and shares lessons learned and advice to help others navigate their own journey with the condition.

Testimonials from Gastroparesis Patients

1. Emma's Journey
   - Background: Emma was diagnosed with gastroparesis five years ago after experiencing persistent nausea and abdominal pain. Initially,

she struggled with finding the right diet and managing her symptoms.

- Experience: Emma shares how adjusting her diet and incorporating small, frequent meals helped her regain control over her symptoms. She emphasizes the importance of patience and persistence in finding what works best for each individual.

- Quote: "It took time to find the right balance, but now I'm able to manage my symptoms better. The key is to listen to your body and be flexible with your approach."

2. James' Story

- Background: James, a busy professional, faced significant challenges in balancing work and managing gastroparesis. He found it difficult to maintain his diet while traveling for work.

- Experience: James discusses how planning ahead and preparing gastroparesis-friendly snacks for travel helped him manage his condition more effectively. He also highlights the importance of open communication with his employer about his needs.

- Quote: "Preparation is everything. By planning my meals and snacks, I was able to handle work travel without compromising my health."

3. Sophia's Experience
  - Background: Sophia, a college student, had to adjust her lifestyle and social activities to accommodate her gastroparesis. She struggled with feeling isolated and frustrated.
  - Experience: Sophia talks about how joining a support group helped her connect with others who understood her struggles. She also shares how she adapted her social life by communicating her needs to friends and finding new ways to participate in activities.
  - Quote: "Joining a support group made a huge difference. It's comforting to know that others are going through the same thing and to share advice and encouragement."

4. Liam's Perspective
  - Background: Liam, a retired veteran, was diagnosed with gastroparesis later in life. He

initially found it challenging to adjust to dietary changes and manage symptoms alongside other health conditions.

- Experience: Liam emphasizes the importance of maintaining a positive attitude and staying engaged in hobbies and interests. He also shares how working closely with his healthcare team helped him manage his condition more effectively.

- Quote: "Staying positive and involved in activities I enjoy has been crucial. Don't let gastroparesis define you—focus on what you can control and keep moving forward."

Lessons Learned and Advice

1. Find What Works for You:
   - Personalization: Each person with gastroparesis may have different triggers and tolerances. Experiment with various dietary adjustments, medications, and lifestyle changes to find what works best for you.
   - Flexibility: Be prepared to adapt your strategies as needed. What works today may

need to be adjusted in the future based on changes in your condition or lifestyle.

2. Prioritize Self-Care:
   - Self-Awareness: Pay attention to your body's signals and adjust your routine accordingly. Regular self-care and self-compassion are essential for managing chronic conditions.
   - Balance: Strive to balance managing your condition with maintaining a fulfilling and enjoyable life. Engage in activities that bring you joy and relaxation.

3. Build a Support Network:
   - Seek Support: Connect with others who have gastroparesis through support groups, online communities, or local organizations. Sharing experiences and advice can provide comfort and practical tips.
   - Communicate: Keep your friends, family, and healthcare providers informed about your needs and experiences. Open communication can foster understanding and support.

4. Stay Informed:

- Education: Continuously educate yourself about gastroparesis and new management strategies. Knowledge empowers you to make informed decisions about your health and treatment.

- Resource Utilization: Utilize resources such as books, websites, and healthcare professionals to stay updated on effective management techniques.

5. Embrace a Positive Mindset:

- Resilience: Cultivate resilience and a positive outlook. While living with gastroparesis can be challenging, maintaining a hopeful and proactive attitude can improve your quality of life.

- Celebrate Progress: Acknowledge and celebrate small victories and improvements in your condition. Recognizing progress can boost your morale and motivation.

These personal stories and lessons offer valuable perspectives and advice for those living with gastroparesis. By learning from others' experiences and applying practical strategies, you can better navigate the challenges of managing the condition and enhance your overall well-being.

Conclusion

Living with gastroparesis presents unique challenges, but with the right strategies and support, it is possible to manage symptoms effectively and maintain a fulfilling life. This guide has covered a broad spectrum of topics to help you understand, manage, and adapt to gastroparesis, including:

- - Understanding Gastroparesis: From its definition and causes to its impact on daily life, gaining a comprehensive understanding of gastroparesis is the first step toward effective management.
- - Managing Gastroparesis: Practical advice on medical treatments, dietary management, lifestyle adjustments, and symptom monitoring helps you navigate daily challenges and make informed decisions.
- - Recipes for Gastroparesis Relief: Enjoying a variety of safe and nutritious

meals and snacks can contribute to symptom relief and overall well-being.

- - Tips and Strategies for Daily Living: Learn how to handle social situations, travel, and build a supportive network to enhance your quality of life.
- - Personal Stories and Experiences: Real-life testimonials offer inspiration and practical insights from those who have faced similar challenges.

By combining medical knowledge with personal experiences and self-care practices, you can develop a holistic approach to managing gastroparesis. Remember that each person's journey is unique, and finding the right balance may take time. Stay informed, seek support, and be patient with yourself as you navigate the complexities of living with this condition.

Ultimately, embracing a proactive and informed approach can help you lead a healthier, more satisfying life despite the challenges of gastroparesis. Your journey is a testament to resilience and adaptability, and with the right tools and support, you can thrive in your personal and daily endeavors.

www.ingramcontent.com/pod-product-compliance
Lightning Source LLC
Chambersburg PA
CBHW050815250726

48653CB00006B/2246